DIABETES MANAGEMENT GUIDE

"Achieving Balance & Wellness with Diabetes: A Step-by-Step Guide to Taking Charge of Your Health"

AUSTIN TRIUMPH

Copyright © 2023 by AUSTIN TRIUMPH.

All rights reserved. No part of this book may be reproduced, scanned, or distributed in any printed or electronic form without permission from the author.

Please do not participate in or encourage piracy of copyrighted materials in violation of the author's rights. Purchase only authorized editions.

Table of Contents

I. INTRODUCTION

Once upon a time, there was a man named Bob who had suffered from diabetes for a long time. He had been diagnosed with the condition at a young age, and had been struggling to manage it ever since.

Bob took his medication religiously and followed the instructions of his doctor to the letter, but his diabetes still seemed to be getting worse. He was constantly tired and unable to focus, and had to take regular breaks from work to rest.

His diet was restricted and he had to watch everything he ate, making it hard to enjoy the foods he once loved. At some point, Bob's diabetes had become so severe that he had to start taking insulin injections.

The daily injections were painful and inconvenient, and he was afraid of what the future held for him.

One day, Bob went to the doctor for a check-up. After a thorough examination, the doctor told him that his diabetes was finally under control.

He was relieved and ecstatic to hear the news. Bob was determined to make the most of his newfound health. He changed his diet, exercised regularly and began to take a more active role in managing his condition.

He was surprised to find that he had more energy than he had in years and felt like a new person. Bob was thankful for the second chance he had been given and was determined to make the most of it.

He was grateful for the support of his family and friends and was determined to stay healthy and happy.

This is the story of Bob, a man who suffered from diabetes for a long time but eventually found the strength, zeal and knowlodge to overcome it and live a fuller life.

Diabetes is a chronic metabolic disorder that affects the way the body processes glucose, or blood sugar.

It is characterized by high blood sugar levels, which can cause a variety of complications over time.

There are two main types of diabetes: type 1 and type 2.

Type 1 diabetes is an autoimmune disorder where the body does not produce enough insulin, while type 2 diabetes is when the body does not properly use the insulin it produces.

Both types can be managed with lifestyle changes and medication.

Definition of Diabetes:

Diabetes is a chronic condition characterized by high levels of glucose in the blood, either due to defects in insulin production or an inability to utilize insulin properly.

It is a leading cause of heart disease, stroke, kidney disease, blindness, and other health problems.

The two main types of diabetes are type 1 diabetes, which is caused by an autoimmune destruction of the beta cells of the pancreas that normally produce insulin, and type 2 diabetes, which is caused by insulin resistance, a condition in which the body does not respond normally to the insulin it produces.

According to the World Health Organization, in 2019, 463 million adults (20-79 years) were living with diabetes, and this number is projected to increase to 578 million by 2030. An estimated 1.6 million deaths are directly attributed to diabetes each year, and it is the seventh leading cause of death worldwide. Diabetes is a major cause of blindness, kidney failure, heart attack, stroke and lower limb amputation.

 In 2016, an estimated US$1.2 trillion was spent on diabetes and its complications.

In 2019, an estimated 88 million adults aged 18-99 years had diabetes in the WHO African Region. This is projected to increase to 130 million by 2045.

As of 2019, an estimated 39 million women aged 18-99 years had diabetes in the WHO African Region. This is projected to increase to 54 million by 2045.

In 2019, an estimated 131 million adults aged 18-99 years had diabetes in the WHO South-East Asia Region. This is projected to increase to 173 million by 2045. As of 2019, an estimated 58 million women aged 18-99 years had diabetes in the WHO South-East Asia Region. This is projected to increase to 77 million by 2045.

In 2019, an estimated 221 million adults aged 18-99 years had diabetes in the WHO European Region. This is projected to increase to 250 million by 2045. As of 2019, an estimated 94 million women aged 18-99 years had diabetes in the WHO European Region. This is projected to increase to 106 million by 2045.

Types of Diabetes:

There are two main types of diabetes

- type 1 diabetes and type 2 diabetes.

Type 1 diabetes is an autoimmune disorder in which the body's immune system attacks and destroys the insulin-producing beta cells of the pancreas.

Without insulin, the body is unable to use glucose for energy, so blood glucose levels become elevated.

This type of diabetes is usually diagnosed in children and young adults, and it accounts for about 10% of all diabetes cases.

Type 2 diabetes is a metabolic disorder in which the body either does not produce enough insulin or does not respond properly to the insulin it produces.

As a result, glucose builds up in the blood instead of being used by the cells for energy. Type 2 diabetes is typically diagnosed in adults, but it is increasingly being seen in children and adolescents, and it accounts for about 90% of all diabetes cases.

Both type 1 and type 2 diabetes can be managed through lifestyle modifications, such as exercise and diet, and with medication. It is important to consult with a healthcare provider for the best treatment plan for each individual.

Symptoms of Diabetes:

1. **Increased thirst and urination:** People with diabetes may experience an increase in thirst, needing to urinate more often than usual (especially at night).

2. **Weight loss:** Diabetes can cause unexpected weight loss due to the body's inability to properly process glucose, leading to the body burning its own muscle and fat for energy.

3. **Fatigue:** Fatigue and tiredness can be caused by high blood sugar levels, which can interfere with normal sleep patterns and make a person feel tired during the day.

4. **Blurred vision:** High blood sugar can cause changes in the shape of the lens of the eye, leading to blurred vision.

5. **Slow-healing sores or frequent infections**: High blood sugar can impair the body's natural healing process, making it difficult for wounds to heal and making the person more susceptible to infections.

.

6. **Numbness or tingling in the hands and feet:** High blood sugar can damage the nerves, leading to numbness, tingling, or pain in the hands and feet.

7. **Unusual smells on the body:** Diabetes can cause a sweet or fruity smell on the person's breath, due to high levels of ketones in the blood.

8. **Cuts, bruises, or sores that don't heal:** High blood sugar can slow the body's natural healing process and make it difficult for wounds to heal

II. DIAGNOSIS

Diagnosis is the process of determining the cause of a condition, symptom, or illness based on a thorough evaluation of the patient's medical history, physical examination, and other diagnostic tests.

It involves identifying a disease or condition based on signs and symptoms, laboratory tests, or other procedures. It is an important part of the medical process and helps to inform the treatment plan.

DIABETIC DIAGNOSIS:

A diagnosis of diabetes is typically based on two tests: the fasting plasma glucose (FPG) test and the oral glucose tolerance test (OGTT).

The FPG test measures your blood glucose level after you have fasted for at least 8 hours. The OGTT measures your blood glucose level after you have been given a sugary drink.

Diagnosis can also be made using the A1C test, which measures your average blood glucose level over the past 2-3 months.

The A1C test is not used to diagnose diabetes, but it can be used to confirm a diagnosis and monitor your treatment.

Other tests that may be used to diagnose diabetes include urine tests to detect high levels of glucose, a C-peptide test to measure C-peptide levels (a protein released with insulin), and a test to measure antibodies that your body may produce if it has developed an autoimmune response to insulin.

Your doctor may also take an individualized approach to diagnosis, considering your age, race/ethnicity, family history, physical activity, and other factors.

UNDERSTANDING YOUR DIAGNOSIS:

It is important for those who are at risk of developing diabetes to understand their diagnosis, so they can take the necessary steps to manage their condition.

The first step to understanding a diabetic diagnosis is to be familiar with the different types of diabetes. Type 1 diabetes is an autoimmune disorder in which the body does not produce enough insulin, while type 2 diabetes is a condition in which the body does not respond properly to insulin. Knowing the type of diabetes a person has can help them understand how to manage it.

The next step is to understand the risk factors associated with developing diabetes.

These risk factors include age, family history, obesity, physical inactivity, and a sedentary lifestyle. Understanding these risk factors can help people make lifestyle changes that can reduce their risk of developing diabetes.

t is also important to understand the symptoms of diabetes, as this can help people identify the condition early. Common symptoms include excessive thirst, frequent urination, extreme hunger, fatigue, and blurred vision. Knowing these symptoms can help people get the necessary medical care as soon as possible.

Finally, it is important for people to understand the importance of regular medical care once they have been diagnosed with diabetes.

This includes regular blood sugar monitoring, check-ups with the doctor, and following any recommended lifestyle modifications. Working with a healthcare provider is the best way to ensure that diabetes is managed properly and that long-term health complications are minimized.

By understanding their diabetic diagnosis, those who are at risk of developing diabetes can take the necessary steps to manage their condition and reduce their risk of developing long-term health   complications.

III. TREATMENT

MONITORING DIABETES:

Monitoring diabetes is an important part of managing this condition. The most common way to do so is to use a glucometer or blood glucose monitor.

This device measures your blood sugar level. You should check your blood sugar before meals, two hours after meals, and at bedtime. It is recommended to keep a log of all results and compare them to the target range set by your doctor.

Other methods for monitoring diabetes include regular check-ups with your doctor, tracking your diet and activity level, and monitoring your weight. During your visits to the doctor, your doctor will take a physical exam and review your blood tests and A1C levels. A1C is a test that measures your average blood sugar level over the past two to three months.

Your doctor may also order other tests to check your organ health and blood lipid levels.

When it comes to diet and activity level, it is important to make healthy choices. Eating a balanced diet, exercising regularly, and avoiding smoking and excessive alcohol intake can help you to manage your diabetes.

Keeping track of your food and activity can help you to make sure that you are staying within healthy ranges.

Finally, weight management is a critical factor in managing diabetes. Gaining or losing too much weight can cause your diabetes to become more difficult to manage. You should aim to keep your weight within a healthy range.

Monitoring your diabetes is an important part of managing the condition.

By regularly checking your blood sugar, visiting your doctor, tracking your diet and activity level, and maintaining a healthy weight, you can better manage your diabetes and reduce your risk of complications.

MEDICATIONS FOR DIABETES:

1. **Insulin:** This is a hormone produced by the pancreas that helps the body use glucose for energy. It is the main medication used to treat type 1 diabetes and can also be used to treat type 2 diabetes.

2. **Metformin:** This is an oral medication that helps reduce blood glucose levels by decreasing the amount of glucose produced by the liver and increasing the sensitivity of the body's cells to insulin.

3. **Sulfonylureas:** This class of drugs stimulates the pancreas to produce more insulin, which helps the body use glucose more effectively.

4. **GLP-1 Receptor Agonists:** This class of drugs helps the body produce more insulin in response to rising blood glucose levels.

5. **Thiazolidinediones**: This class of drugs helps increase the body's sensitivity to insulin, which helps the body use glucose more effectively.

6. **DPP-4 Inhibitors:** This class of drugs helps the body to produce more insulin and reduce the amount of glucose the body absorbs from food.

7. **Amylin Analogs:** This class of drugs helps slow the absorption of glucose from food, which helps keep blood glucose levels stable.

8. **Alpha-glucosidase Inhibitors:** This class of drugs helps slow the digestion and absorption of carbohydrates in the body, which helps keep blood glucose levels stable.

9. **Bile Acid Sequestrants:** This class of drugs helps reduce the amount of glucose absorbed from the intestines, which helps keep blood glucose levels stable.

10. **Meglitinides:** This class of drugs helps the pancreas produce more insulin in response to rising blood glucose levels.

INSULIN ADMINISTRATION:

When it comes to insulin administration, there are several different types of insulin available and the type that is chosen will depend on the individual's needs.

Rapid-acting insulin is designed to be taken before meals and it works quickly to lower blood sugar levels.

Long-acting insulin is intended to be taken once or twice a day, and it helps to keep blood sugar levels steady throughout the day. Intermediate-acting insulin is usually taken twice a day, and it helps to maintain blood sugar levels between meals.

When taking insulin injections, it is important to follow the instructions provided by your doctor.

It is important to inject the insulin into the correct area of the body, as each type of insulin is designed to work best when injected in a certain area.

It is important to inject the insulin into the correct area of the body, as each type of insulin is designed to work best when injected in a certain area.

This could include the abdomen, thigh, arm, or buttocks. It is also important to ensure that the insulin is injected at the right time and at the right dose.

Insulin administration can help to manage diabetes, but it is important to follow the instructions provided by your doctor. It is also important to monitor blood sugar levels regularly and to make any necessary lifestyle changes to help keep blood sugar levels in check.

IV. NUTRITION

Eating for Diabetes:

Eating for diabetes can be tricky and requires careful planning. A diabetes-friendly diet is one that focuses on whole, unprocessed foods and is low in added sugar, salt, and unhealthy fats.

 Eating a balanced diet of fresh vegetables, fruits, lean proteins, whole grains, and healthy fats can help keep blood sugar levels in check and prevent long-term complications.

When selecting foods, it's important to choose those that are low on the glycemic index, meaning they won't cause a rapid spike in blood sugar levels. Examples of low glycemic foods include oatmeal, quinoa, legumes, and non-starchy vegetables.

It's also important to combine proteins, carbohydrates, and fats at each meal to maintain steady blood sugar levels.

When eating carbohydrates, opt for complex carbs such as whole wheat bread, brown rice, and other whole grains.

Protein sources such as chicken, fish, and beans are also great for stabilizing blood sugar. Healthy fats such as avocados, nuts, and olive oil are also beneficial.

In addition, portion control is an important part of managing diabetes. Eating smaller meals and snacks throughout the day can help keep blood sugar levels steady.

Finally, be sure to include plenty of fiber in your diet. Eating high-fiber foods such as fruits, vegetables, legumes, and whole grains helps to slow down the digestion of carbohydrates, which helps to prevent blood sugar spikes.

Eating a healthy, diabetes-friendly diet can make a huge difference in managing diabetes. Be sure to talk to your doctor or a registered dietitian to learn more about eating for diabetes.

Meal planning and carb Counting:

Meal Planning:

1. Choose a variety of nutrient-dense foods that are low in saturated fat, sodium, and added sugars.

2. Include a balance of fruits and vegetables, lean proteins, whole grains, and low-fat dairy.

3. Plan meals around carbohydrates.

4. Incorporate healthy fats like olive oil, nuts, and avocados.

5. Eat a healthy breakfast and snacks throughout the day.

Carb Counting:

1. Measure and weigh all food to accurately track carbohydrates.

2. Follow a consistent meal plan.

3. Count the carbohydrates in each food item that you consume.

4. Include carb-containing foods in each meal and snack.

5. Read food labels to understand the grams of carbohydrates in each food.

6. Adjust insulin doses to match carbohydrate intake.

Recommended meals for Diabetes:

1. Oatmeal with berries

2. Salmon with roasted vegetables

3. Quinoa bowl with beans and vegetables

4. Greek yogurt with nuts and seeds

5. Lentil soup

6. Chickpea curry

7. Egg white omelette

8. Tuna salad wrap

9. Grilled chicken with sweet potato

10. Mixed salad with lean protein

11. Broiled Salmon with Asparagus

12. Edamame

etc.

V. Exercises

1. **Aerobic Exercise:** Aerobic exercise, also known as cardiovascular exercise, is any type of physical activity that increases your heart rate. Examples of aerobic exercise include jogging, swimming, walking, biking, and dancing. This type of exercise can help improve insulin sensitivity, helping your body use insulin more effectively.

2. **Resistance Exercise:** Resistance exercise, such as weight lifting, is any activity that puts stress on your muscles. This type of exercise can help build muscle mass and improve insulin sensitivity.

3. **Yoga:** Yoga is a form of exercise that combines physical poses with deep breathing. Studies have shown that yoga can help improve insulin sensitivity and reduce levels of stress hormones, which can help improve blood sugar control.

4. **High-Intensity Interval Training (HIIT):** HIIT is a type of exercise that involves short bursts of intense activity followed by periods of rest. This type of exercise can help improve insulin sensitivity and reduce blood sugar levels.

5. **Tai Chi:** Tai chi is a form of exercise that involves slow, gentle movements that promote balance, flexibility, and relaxation. Studies have shown that tai chi can help reduce stress and improve insulin sensitivity.

6. **Walking:** Walking is a great form of exercise for people with diabetes. It is low impact, easy to do, and can be done almost anywhere. Studies have shown that walking can help reduce blood sugar levels and improve insulin sensitivity.

VI. MANAGING OTHER CONDITIONS

Hypoglycemia:

Hypoglycemia is a condition where the body has a low level of blood sugar, usually below 70 mg/dL.

It can occur when the body doesn't have enough glucose, or when the body's cells don't use the glucose that is present. Symptoms of hypoglycemia can include sweating, dizziness, confusion, hunger, weakness, and rapid heartbeat.

To manage hypoglycemia, it is important to eat small, frequent meals that include complex carbohydrates, lean proteins, and healthy fats.

It is also important to avoid sugary snacks and drinks. If hypoglycemia is severe, a doctor may prescribe medication to help regulate blood sugar levels. Exercising regularly and getting adequate sleep can also help to manage and prevent hypoglycemia.

Hyperglycemia:

Hyperglycemia is a condition in which an individual has an elevated blood glucose (blood sugar) level.

It is typically seen in people with diabetes, when the body does not produce enough insulin or does not use it properly.

To manage hyperglycemia, people should adjust their diet to reduce sugar and carbohydrates, exercise regularly, and monitor their blood glucose levels.

Some individuals may need to take medications to help control their blood sugar levels.

It is important to speak with a doctor or healthcare professional to devise an appropriate plan to manage hyperglycemia.

VII. MENTAL HEALTH

Maintaining mental health while living with diabetes can be a challenge, but it is important to prioritize self-care in order to manage stress and anxiety. Here are some tips to help you stay mentally healthy while dealing with diabetes:

COPING WITH DIABETES

1. **Connect with Others:** Connecting with other people who understand what it is like to live with diabetes can provide valuable support. Consider joining a diabetes support group or participating in online forums to connect with others in a similar situation.

2. **Take Time for Yourself:** Make sure to take time each day to do something that you enjoy and that helps you relax. This could be anything from meditating to going for a walk in nature.

3. **Eat Healthy:** Eating a healthy diet can help you manage your blood sugar levels and give you energy to manage stress. Make sure to include plenty of fruits, vegetables, whole grains, lean proteins, and healthy fats in your meals.

4. Exercise Regularly: Exercise not only helps to regulate blood sugar levels, but it also releases endorphins that can help reduce stress and anxiety. Consider taking a yoga class or going for a jog to get your body moving.

5. **Get Enough Sleep:** Poor sleep can increase stress and make managing diabetes more difficult.

TALKING WITH A DOCTOR

1. **Prepare for your appointment:**
Make a list of questions, concerns, and symptoms you want to discuss with your doctor. Also, bring a list of all the medications you are taking.

2. **Be honest and open:**
Talk openly and honestly about your symptoms and any lifestyle changes you've made to manage your diabetes.

3. **Clarify any of the doctor's instructions:**
If there's anything you don't understand or need more information on, make sure to ask.

4. **Take notes:**
Write down any new information or instructions that your doctor gives you.

5. **Ask for a follow-up:**
Ask for a follow-up appointment if you need one.

6. **Follow up with your doctor:**
Don't be afraid to call or email your doctor if you need help or have additional questions.

VIII. RESOURCES

Support groups are a type of group therapy where people who have similar issues or experiences come together to share their stories, provide emotional support to one another, and learn coping strategies.

Support groups are typically facilitated by a qualified mental health professional and may be focused on a particular issue, such as bereavement, addiction, or mental illness.

BENEFITS OF SUPPORT GROUPS

1. **Exchange of information and ideas:** Support groups allow diabetics to exchange information, ask questions, and have access to a variety of helpful resources and tips. This can help diabetics learn more about their condition and how to manage it effectively.

2. **Sense of community:** Being part of a support group can provide a sense of community that can be very comforting and reassuring. It can help diabetics feel less isolated and more connected to others who are dealing with the same   condition.

3. Emotional support:

Support groups can provide emotional support and understanding that can be invaluable to diabetics. This can include listening to stories, sharing experiences, and offering encouragement.

4. Improved quality of life:

Studies have shown that support groups can help diabetics improve their quality of life. This can include better management of the disease, improved coping skills, and increased self-confidence.

5. Access to professionals:

Support groupscan provide access to professionals such as nurses, dietitians, and doctors who are knowledgeable about diabetes. This can be incredibly helpful in providing advice and guidance.

IX. CONCLUSION

TIPS FOR LONG-TERM MANAGEMENT:

.1. Establish a routine for monitoring blood sugar levels and regular medical checkups.

2. Follow a healthy diet with plenty of vegetables, fruits, and whole grains.

3. Exercise regularly to help keep your blood sugar levels in check.

4. Manage stress in healthy ways, such as through yoga, meditation, or counseling.

5. Quit smoking if you are a smoker.

6. Be aware of the signs and symptoms of hypoglycemia and hyperglycemia and how to treat them.

7. Take your medications as prescribed.

.

8. Monitor your feet regularly for signs of infection or other problems.

9. Make sure you are up to date on all recommended vaccinations.

10. Stay connected with your healthcare team for regular monitoring and support

IN CONCLUSION

Diabetes management is about taking control of your health and destiny, and the rewards are great.

With the knowledge and tools you've acquired from this book, you can now confidently make informed decisions and take the necessary steps to enjoy a healthier, happier and more fulfilling life.

So, take charge of your diabetes today, and you'll be one step closer to achieving your goals and living life to the fullest!

References:

U.S. Department of Health and Human Services. (2018). Your Guide to Diabetes: Type 1 and Type 2.

-https://www.niddk.nih.gov/health-information/diabetes/overview/what-is-diabetes

World health Organization
--https://www.who.int/

images credit : pixabay

www.ingramcontent.com/pod-product-compliance
Lightning Source LLC
Chambersburg PA
CBHW060849260726
48661CB00002B/688